Personal Details

Type of Animal _____

Breed _____

Name _____

Birth date _____

Current Age _____

Owner Details

Name _____

Contact no. _____

Email _____

Notes

Vaccination Record

Date	Age	Vaccine	Brand	Batch#	Vet

Notes

Vaccination Record

Date	Age	Vaccine	Brand	Batch#	Vet

Notes

Vaccination Record

Date	Age	Vaccine	Brand	Batch#	Vet

Notes

Vaccination Record

Date	Age	Vaccine	Brand	Batch#	Vet

Notes

Vaccination Record

Date	Age	Vaccine	Brand	Batch#	Vet

Notes

Vaccination Record

Date	Age	Vaccine	Brand	Batch#	Vet

Notes

Vaccination Record

Date	Age	Vaccine	Brand	Batch#	Vet

Notes

Vaccination Record

Date	Age	Vaccine	Brand	Batch#	Vet

Notes

Vaccination Record

Date	Age	Vaccine	Brand	Batch#	Vet

Notes

Vaccination Record

Date	Age	Vaccine	Brand	Batch#	Vet

Notes

Vaccination Record

Date	Age	Vaccine	Brand	Batch#	Vet

Notes

Vaccination Record

Date	Age	Vaccine	Brand	Batch#	Vet

Notes

Vaccination Record

Date	Age	Vaccine	Brand	Batch#	Vet

Notes

Vaccination Record

Date	Age	Vaccine	Brand	Batch#	Vet

Notes

Vaccination Record

Date	Age	Vaccine	Brand	Batch#	Vet

Notes

Vaccination Record

Date	Age	Vaccine	Brand	Batch#	Vet

Notes

Vaccination Record

Date	Age	Vaccine	Brand	Batch#	Vet

Notes

Vaccination Record

Date	Age	Vaccine	Brand	Batch#	Vet

Notes

Vaccination Record

Date	Age	Vaccine	Brand	Batch#	Vet

Notes

Vaccination Record

Date	Age	Vaccine	Brand	Batch#	Vet

Notes

Vaccination Record

Date	Age	Vaccine	Brand	Batch#	Vet

Notes

Vaccination Record

Date	Age	Vaccine	Brand	Batch#	Vet

Notes

Vaccination Record

Date	Age	Vaccine	Brand	Batch#	Vet

Notes

Vaccination Record

Date	Age	Vaccine	Brand	Batch#	Vet

Notes

Vaccination Record

Date	Age	Vaccine	Brand	Batch#	Vet

Notes

Vaccination Record

Date	Age	Vaccine	Brand	Batch#	Vet

Notes

Vaccination Record

Date	Age	Vaccine	Brand	Batch#	Vet

Notes

Vaccination Record

Date	Age	Vaccine	Brand	Batch#	Vet

Notes

Vaccination Record

Date	Age	Vaccine	Brand	Batch#	Vet

Notes

Vaccination Record

Date	Age	Vaccine	Brand	Batch#	Vet

Notes

Vaccination Record

Date	Age	Vaccine	Brand	Batch#	Vet

Notes

Vaccination Record

Date	Age	Vaccine	Brand	Batch#	Vet

Notes

Vaccination Record

Date	Age	Vaccine	Brand	Batch#	Vet

Notes

Vaccination Record

Date	Age	Vaccine	Brand	Batch#	Vet

Notes

Vaccination Record

Date	Age	Vaccine	Brand	Batch#	Vet

Notes

Vaccination Record

Date	Age	Vaccine	Brand	Batch#	Vet

Notes

Vaccination Record

Date	Age	Vaccine	Brand	Batch#	Vet

Notes

Vaccination Record

Date	Age	Vaccine	Brand	Batch#	Vet

Notes

Vaccination Record

Date	Age	Vaccine	Brand	Batch#	Vet

Notes

Vaccination Record

Date	Age	Vaccine	Brand	Batch#	Vet

Notes

Vaccination Record

Date	Age	Vaccine	Brand	Batch#	Vet

Notes

Vaccination Record

Date	Age	Vaccine	Brand	Batch#	Vet

Notes

Vaccination Record

Date	Age	Vaccine	Brand	Batch#	Vet

Notes

Vaccination Record

Date	Age	Vaccine	Brand	Batch#	Vet

Notes

Vaccination Record

Date	Age	Vaccine	Brand	Batch#	Vet

Notes

Vaccination Record

Date	Age	Vaccine	Brand	Batch#	Vet

Notes

Vaccination Record

Date	Age	Vaccine	Brand	Batch#	Vet

Notes

Vaccination Record

Date	Age	Vaccine	Brand	Batch#	Vet

Notes

Vaccination Record

Date	Age	Vaccine	Brand	Batch#	Vet

Notes

Vaccination Record

Date	Age	Vaccine	Brand	Batch#	Vet

Notes

Vaccination Record

Date	Age	Vaccine	Brand	Batch#	Vet

Notes

Vaccination Record

Date	Age	Vaccine	Brand	Batch#	Vet

Notes

Vaccination Record

Date	Age	Vaccine	Brand	Batch#	Vet

Notes

Vaccination Record

Date	Age	Vaccine	Brand	Batch#	Vet

www.ingramcontent.com/pod-product-compliance
Lightning Source LLC
Chambersburg PA
CBHW070421220526
45466CB00004B/1499